LOW POTASSIUM

COOKBOOK: A DIET

PLAN FOR BEGINNERS

AND SENIORS

A Simple Guide to Preventing Kidney

Disease, Promoting Heart Health,

Regulating Blood Pressure, and Preventing

Hyperkalemia

Michael Slowick, RDN

COPYRIGHT PAGE

completeness or accuracy. Any statements made by sales employees or representatives, whether verbal or written, do not constitute extended or implied guarantees.

Table of Contents

CHAPTER I: GETTING FAMILIAR WITH THE LOW POTASSIUM DIET

Insufficient levels of potassium in the bloodstream, medically termed as hypokalemia, pose significant risks to the optimal functioning of various bodily systems, including neurons, muscles, and notably, the heart muscle. This mineral plays a pivotal role in maintaining the electrical conductivity necessary for proper nerve transmission and muscle contraction, particularly crucial for the heart's rhythmic activity.

The intricate balance of potassium in the body is primarily regulated by the kidneys, which work diligently to eliminate excess potassium through urine and sweat. However, when this balance is disrupted, either due to inadequate intake or excessive loss, the repercussions can be profound.

In cases of severe hypokalemia, the disruptions to cardiac rhythm, known as arrhythmias, can lead to life-threatening complications. Additionally, pronounced muscular weakness can impair everyday functions and, in extreme scenarios, result in paralysis. Conversely, individuals experiencing mild hypokalemia may exhibit no outward symptoms, making it a silent but potentially hazardous condition.

Addressing hypokalemia necessitates a multifaceted approach involving dietary adjustments, medical interventions, and vigilant monitoring. Collaboration with healthcare professionals is paramount, as they can provide tailored guidance to ensure adequate potassium intake through diet and, when necessary, supplementation.

Moreover, prompt medical attention is imperative for those experiencing prolonged vomiting or diarrhea, as these conditions can exacerbate potassium depletion. Recognizing the severity of hypokalemia is crucial, as more serious cases may require intravenous administration of potassium to swiftly restore levels to a safe range.

Regular follow-up appointments with healthcare providers are indispensable for monitoring progress and adjusting treatment plans as needed. Through comprehensive management strategies and ongoing medical oversight, individuals can effectively mitigate the risks associated with hypokalemia and safeguard their overall well-being.

What exactly constitutes hypokalemia?

When the concentration of potassium in your bloodstream falls below the normal range, a medical condition known as hypokalemia arises, posing potential health risks. Typically, the average adult maintains a potassium concentration within the range of 3.5 to 5.2 milliequivalents per liter (mEq/L) or millimoles per liter (mmol/L). However, severe hypokalemia is diagnosed when levels plummet below 3 mEq/L (3 mmol/L), signifying a critical imbalance.

Electrolytes such as potassium carry a slight electric charge when dissolved in bodily fluids. This mineral is indispensable for the proper functioning of muscles, nerve cells, and overall cellular health. Primarily sourced from dietary intake, potassium intake is regulated by the kidneys, which excrete any excess through urine to maintain optimal levels within the body.

The significance of potassium as a nutrient cannot be overstated, as it plays multifaceted roles in ensuring the vitality of muscles, neurons, and cardiac function. Additionally, it contributes to the efficient operation of the digestive system and fosters skeletal strength. Insufficient potassium levels can lead to disruptions in nerve signal transmission, irregular heart rhythms, muscle weakness, and in severe cases, paralysis.

Thus, understanding the critical role of maintaining adequate potassium levels is paramount for safeguarding one's health and overall well-being. Prioritizing dietary choices and mindful monitoring of potassium intake can help mitigate the risks associated with hypokalemia, ensuring optimal physiological functioning and vitality.

Factors leading to Hypokalemia

The human body operates like a finely tuned orchestra, with various systems and organs working in harmony to maintain equilibrium. Among these crucial players are the kidneys, the skin, and the digestive tract, each offering potential pathways for the delicate balance of potassium to be disrupted.

Consider potassium, an essential electrolyte vital for numerous bodily functions, from nerve transmission to muscle contraction. Its levels can be influenced by a myriad of factors, leading to a condition known as hypokalemia, wherein the potassium concentration in the blood falls below normal levels.

One common culprit contributing to hypokalemia is insufficient dietary intake of potassium, compounded by depleted magnesium levels. This deficiency can stem from various sources, including preexisting medical conditions or the use of prescribed medications.

Digging deeper, we find that excessive potassium losses through the digestive tract often shoulder the blame for decreased circulating levels. This depletion may arise from frequent laxative use, chronic vomiting episodes, or persistent diarrhea, all of which can strip the body of its potassium reserves.

Yet, the web of causality surrounding hypokalemia extends far beyond these primary factors. For instance, individuals grappling with eating disorders like bulimia nervosa may disrupt their potassium balance. Similarly, profuse sweating, a condition known as hyperhidrosis, can lead to potassium loss, as can alcohol use disorder.

The pharmacological realm also plays a significant role in perturbing potassium levels. Diuretic medications, designed to increase urine output, can inadvertently flush potassium from the body. Likewise, drugs like insulin, certain antibiotics, and corticosteroids may throw potassium regulation off-kilter.

Moreover, underlying medical conditions such as adrenal illnesses (e.g., primary aldosteronism, Cushing's syndrome) and chronic renal disease can predispose individuals to hypokalemia. Hypomagnesemia, characterized by low magnesium levels, further exacerbates the potassium imbalance.

Even rarer genetic disorders, such as Bartter's syndrome and Gitelman syndrome, disrupt potassium regulation at a systemic level. Additionally, illnesses like Liddle syndrome, though exceedingly uncommon, underscore the diverse array of factors that can contribute to potassium abnormalities.

In the labyrinthine landscape of diagnosing and treating hypokalemia, understanding its multifaceted origins is paramount. Only by unraveling the intricate interplay of dietary, pharmacological, and physiological factors can healthcare providers effectively address potassium imbalances and restore equilibrium to the body's electrolyte composition.

Signs of Hypokalemia

Hypokalemia, a condition characterized by a blood potassium level below 3.5 mmol per liter, underscores the critical role of potassium in sustaining bodily functions. Potassium serves as a linchpin in the orchestration of muscular contractions, facilitation of normal neuronal activities, and regulation of fluid balance within the body. Despite its significance, the contemporary dietary patterns prevalent in Western societies often fall short in providing adequate potassium intake, primarily due to the predominant consumption of processed foods at the expense of potassium-rich whole plant foods such as fruits, vegetables, legumes, and nuts.

Nutritional deficiencies constitute one facet contributing to hypokalemia, yet an array of other factors also weigh in, including fluid loss, malnutrition, shock, medication usage, and various medical conditions such as renal failure. The initial manifestations of potassium deficiency typically manifest as weakness and fatigue, which stem from diverse physiological mechanisms. Diminished potassium levels impede effective muscular contractions, thereby exacerbating muscle weakness, while also impairing nutrient utilization, leading to lethargy, particularly when insulin synthesis is compromised, culminating in elevated blood glucose levels and diminished cellular energy derived from glucose.

Muscular weakness and cramping often accompany potassium deficiency due to its pivotal role in facilitating neural communication between the brain and skeletal muscles. Depressed potassium levels impede the rapid transmission of nerve impulses, resulting in prolonged muscle contractions and discomforting cramps. Moreover, severe hypokalemia precipitates rhabdomyolysis, a grave condition characterized by muscle breakdown and the release of harmful proteins into circulation, potentially culminating in organ damage if left untreated. Notably, even milder forms of hypokalemia can provoke significant muscular impairment.

Digestive disturbances can ensue from potassium insufficiency, with implications ranging from weakened intestinal contractions to sluggish food transit, fostering conditions like bloating and constipation, particularly pronounced in severe hypokalemia cases. Potassium's significance extends to cardiovascular health, where its regulation within cardiac cells governs the rhythmicity of heart muscle contractions. Disturbances in potassium balance can precipitate cardiac arrhythmias, necessitating prompt medical intervention upon the onset of anomalous heart rhythms.

Furthermore, profound potassium depletion can impinge upon respiratory function, impeding the coordinated expansion and contraction of lung tissue essential for breathing. In severe cases, this deficiency can culminate in respiratory failure, emphasizing the criticality of maintaining adequate potassium levels for sustaining pulmonary integrity. Hospitalized patients with hypokalemia or hyperkalemia exhibit an increased propensity for respiratory compromise, often necessitating mechanical ventilation to sustain respiratory function.

While paresthesia traditionally associates with elevated potassium levels, it can also manifest in individuals afflicted by potassium deficiency, attributable to its pivotal role in preserving normative nerve function. Paresthesia, characterized by tingling or numbness predominantly in the extremities, warrants medical evaluation, especially if enduring or inexplicable by transient factors.

Potassium deficiency can impair renal function, compromising the kidneys' ability to concentrate urine and regulate electrolyte balance, precipitating polyuria and polydipsia. Excessive urinary output coupled with heightened thirst underscores the need for medical assessment to preempt further potassium depletion. Moreover, potassium exerts a modulatory influence on blood pressure regulation, with inadequate dietary intake exacerbating hypertension by thwarting the kidneys' capacity to expel surplus sodium. Proactively ensuring sufficient potassium intake may thus confer benefits in maintaining optimal blood pressure levels, particularly pertinent for individuals predisposed to hypertension, necessitating vigilant medical oversight.

Hypokalemia underscores the multifaceted implications of potassium insufficiency, ranging from neuromuscular dysfunction to cardiovascular and respiratory compromise, necessitating comprehensive management strategies encompassing dietary interventions and medical surveillance to mitigate adverse outcomes.

CHAPTER II: IMPORTANCE OF MINERALS

Minerals play a pivotal role in the intricate dance of life within our bodies, ensuring that vital processes unfold seamlessly. These essential nutrients are categorized into two main groups: macro-minerals, which the body requires in larger amounts, and micro-minerals, which are needed in trace amounts but are no less crucial for optimal health.

Macro-minerals like calcium, potassium, sodium, phosphorus, sulfur, and magnesium are often in the spotlight, but their lesser-known counterparts, the trace minerals, are equally indispensable. Iron, zinc, copper, selenium, fluoride, manganese, and iodine may be needed in smaller quantities, but they wield significant influence over various bodily functions.

Consider iron, for instance, a trace mineral vital for the synthesis of hemoglobin, the oxygen-carrying component of red blood cells. Its absence can lead to anemia, hindering growth and development. Similarly, zinc, another trace mineral, acts as a catalyst for numerous enzymatic reactions, aids in immune function, and promotes wound healing.

These minerals, whether macro or trace, are not just passive spectators in our biological theater; they are integral to the script, influencing everything from the contraction of muscles to the firing of neurons. Sodium, for example, regulates fluid balance and supports muscle function, while potassium ensures proper nerve transmission and cardiac rhythm.

The significance of maintaining adequate mineral levels cannot be overstated. Deficiencies can manifest in various ways, from impaired bone health due to insufficient calcium intake to compromised immune function stemming from zinc deficiency. Moreover, fluctuations in mineral levels can have far-reaching consequences, contributing to conditions such as hypertension or irregular heart rhythms.

Thankfully, a well-rounded diet typically provides the necessary array of minerals. Fruits, vegetables, whole grains, dairy products, and lean meats offer a cornucopia of essential nutrients. However, for those considering mineral supplements, caution is advised. Consulting with a healthcare professional or nutrition expert can ensure that supplementation is tailored to individual needs, preventing the risk of excess or imbalance.

Minerals are the silent architects of our biological infrastructure, shaping everything from the strength of our bones to the resilience of our immune system. Embracing a diverse and balanced diet rich in mineral-rich foods lays the foundation for optimal health and vitality, ensuring that our bodies hum along harmoniously, guided by the orchestration of these essential nutrients.

Dietary Potassium Levels

Potassium, a vital mineral essential for maintaining optimal bodily function, is abundantly present in a plethora of foods, serving as a pivotal electrolyte. Its role in facilitating the efficient transmission of electrical impulses throughout the body cannot be overstated. These impulses orchestrate a symphony of physiological processes, including but not limited to the regulation of blood pressure, the delicate balance of bodily fluids, the facilitation of muscle contractions, the transmission of nerve signals, the digestion of food, the regulation of heart rhythm, and the maintenance of pH balance.

The inability of the human body to produce its own potassium underscores the critical necessity of incorporating potassium-rich foods and beverages into our diets. However, achieving the ideal balance is imperative, as both deficiency and excess of potassium pose significant health risks. The kidneys emerge as unsung heroes in this narrative, as they diligently regulate blood potassium levels by excreting excess potassium through urine.

While a myriad of fruits, vegetables, and select dairy products serve as excellent dietary sources of potassium, the most effective route for potassium absorption remains through the consumption of well-rounded meals. Beyond the ubiquitous banana, other commendable sources of potassium encompass lean meats, whole grains, legumes, and nuts. For the average individual adhering to a balanced diet, concerns regarding potassium intake are typically unfounded. Nevertheless, individuals with clinically low potassium levels may necessitate supplementation under the guidance of medical professionals. In severe cases, intravenous therapy might be warranted to swiftly restore potassium levels to a state of equilibrium.

Insufficient levels of potassium

Hypokalemia denotes a physiological state characterized by an insufficient level of potassium within the body, which can arise from various underlying medical conditions and lifestyle factors. The depletion of potassium reserves can stem from an array of issues, including but not limited to:

1. Kidney disease, wherein renal dysfunction impairs the body's ability to regulate potassium levels effectively.

2. Prolonged and excessive usage of diuretic medications, which promote the excessive excretion of potassium through urine.

3. Intense perspiration, accompanied by symptoms such as profuse sweating, nausea, and vomiting, leading to potassium loss.

4. Magnesium deficiency, which disrupts the intricate balance between potassium and magnesium ions crucial for cellular function.

5. The utilization of certain antibiotics like carbenicillin and penicillin, which may interfere with potassium absorption or utilization within the body.

The manifestation of hypokalemia can vary depending on the degree of potassium depletion, ranging from subtle symptoms to severe, life-threatening complications. Mild decreases in potassium levels may remain asymptomatic, particularly if the body can restore equilibrium post-activity or following a meal. However, severe deficits in potassium may precipitate alarming indications such as:

- Overwhelming fatigue, indicative of the body's struggle to maintain essential physiological processes.
- Muscle weakness, cramping, or spasms, signaling impaired neuromuscular function due to potassium deficiency.
- Disturbances in cardiac rhythm, potentially culminating in arrhythmias that jeopardize cardiovascular health.

- Gastrointestinal disturbances, including issues with digestion, persistent nausea, or recurrent vomiting, reflecting the systemic impact of potassium imbalance on various bodily systems.

The diagnosis of hypokalemia typically involves a comprehensive evaluation, with blood tests serving as the primary diagnostic tool to assess potassium levels accurately. Additionally, healthcare providers may order an electrocardiogram (ECG) to evaluate cardiac function and an arterial blood gas analysis to ascertain pH levels and further elucidate the extent of metabolic disturbances.

Conversely, hyperkalemia, characterized by elevated potassium levels, can also pose significant health risks, albeit less frequently encountered in healthy individuals. Factors contributing to hyperkalemia encompass diverse etiologies, including:

1. Excessive intake of potassium supplements, surpassing the body's capacity for absorption and utilization.

2. Renal disease or dysfunction, impairing the kidneys' ability to excrete excess potassium efficiently.

3. Prolonged episodes of vigorous physical activity, leading to the release of potassium from skeletal muscle stores.

4. Substance abuse, such as cocaine usage, which may disrupt potassium homeostasis through various mechanisms.

5. The utilization of potassium-sparing diuretics or medications like certain chemotherapy agents, which can elevate potassium levels via distinct pharmacological pathways.

6. Underlying medical conditions such as diabetes or traumatic burns, which may precipitate potassium

release from intracellular compartments into the bloodstream.

Elevated potassium levels can precipitate adverse cardiac events, including potentially life-threatening arrhythmias, necessitating vigilant monitoring and intervention. While individuals with predisposing factors may remain asymptomatic despite mildly elevated potassium levels, routine blood testing remains imperative to detect and mitigate potential complications promptly.

Management strategies for hypo- and hyperkalemia diverge based on the underlying etiology and severity of the condition. In cases of hypokalemia, initial interventions typically involve the administration of potassium supplements to replenish depleted stores, particularly effective in individuals with preserved renal function. Severe hypokalemia accompanied by cardiac arrhythmias may necessitate intravenous (IV) potassium therapy to swiftly restore physiological balance.

Conversely, hyperkalemia management focuses on reducing potassium levels while addressing the underlying cause. Potassium-lowering interventions may encompass dietary modifications, medication adjustments, or renal replacement therapy in severe cases. Potassium-sparing diuretics may be contraindicated in individuals with compromised renal function, necessitating careful consideration and medical supervision.

The management of potassium imbalances necessitates a nuanced understanding of underlying pathophysiological mechanisms and tailored interventions to optimize patient outcomes. Collaborative decision-making involving healthcare professionals and informed patient participation is paramount to ensure safe and effective treatment strategies.

CHAPTER III: MANAGING DEPLETED POTASSIUM

In the management of hypokalemia, the indispensable involvement of healthcare providers is paramount for ensuring effective treatment. The approach to addressing this condition is contingent upon the gravity of the underlying medical ailment.

Primarily, oral potassium supplements emerge as the frontline remedy for mild to severe instances of hypokalemia. However, the complexity of certain cases necessitates adjustments to concurrent medications or the resolution of underlying triggers such as gastrointestinal disturbances like diarrhea, emesis, or even eating disorders.

While advocating for a balanced diet rich in potassium-laden edibles is a cornerstone of preventive healthcare, it often proves insufficient in rectifying hypokalemia. This inadequacy stems from the prevalent form of dietary potassium, predominantly bound with phosphate, which renders it incongruent with the potassium chloride primarily utilized in replenishing deficits. Given that hypokalemia may entail a deficit in chloride as well, supplementation with potassium chloride is judicious for the concurrent correction of both electrolyte imbalances. Effective management typically entails adhering to a daily supplementation regimen ranging from 60-80 mmol over a span of days to weeks, contingent upon medical guidance.

Treatment modalities pivot on the severity of the condition. For milder presentations, healthcare providers frequently opt for oral potassium supplements. Conversely, in more severe manifestations, intravenous (IV) administration of potassium may be imperative. Indications for IV therapy encompass markedly low serum potassium levels, cardiac dysrhythmias attributable to hypokalemia, inadequate response to oral supplementation, or potassium depletion surpassing the body's ability to replace it. Furthermore, clinicians embark on an investigative odyssey to identify and redress any underlying etiologies contributing to the development of hypokalemia.

Of paramount concern is the risk of rebound hyperkalemia, a perilous condition characterized by excessively elevated potassium levels, which underscores the indispensability of vigilant monitoring by healthcare practitioners, especially in severe cases mandating IV therapy. While dietary modifications emphasizing potassium-rich fare are conducive to general health, they often fall short in ameliorating the potassium imbalances underpinning hypokalemia.

Origins of Potassium

Incorporating a variety of foods rich in potassium, such as fruits, vegetables, legumes, and nuts, into your diet is widely acknowledged as beneficial for overall health. However, solely relying on dietary adjustments might not suffice for addressing hypokalemia, a condition characterized by low potassium levels in the blood.

The Recommended Daily Intake (RDI) for potassium underwent revision in 2019 under the auspices of the National Academies of Sciences, Engineering, and Medicine (NASEM). This revision led to the establishment of a new RDI benchmarked at 4,500 milligrams per day for adults. Moreover, the NASEM introduced Sufficient Intake (SI) standards, which consider variations in age and gender. Presently, the recommended dietary allowance (RDA) stands at 2,600 milligrams for women and 3,400 milligrams for men.

Nevertheless, it's crucial to grasp that only a fraction, approximately 85% to 90%, of the potassium ingested from your diet is absorbed by your cells. Hence, the Daily Value (DV) percentage on food labels remains set at 4,700 milligrams, underscoring the importance of this nutrient in maintaining a balanced diet.

To assist in making informed dietary choices, here's a breakdown of potassium-rich foods alongside their serving sizes and the corresponding Daily Value percentages they contribute:

- Half a cup of dried apricots (equivalent to 190 grams) provides 1,100 milligrams of potassium, constituting 23% of the Daily Value.

- Cooked lentils, approximately 198 grams, offer 731 milligrams of potassium, representing around 16% of the DV.

- A cup of cooked acorn squash (205 grams) contains 644 milligrams of potassium, contributing 14% of the DV.

- Canned kidney beans, one cup (260 grams) worth, provide 607 milligrams of potassium, amounting to 13% of the DV.

- A single serving (236 mL) of orange juice supplies 496 milligrams of potassium, contributing 11% to the DV.

- A medium-sized banana (115 grams) offers 422 micrograms of Vitamin C, constituting 9% of the DV.

- A 1-ounce (85 grams) serving of sirloin steak contains 315 milligrams of potassium, contributing 7% to the DV.

- A cup of 1% fat milk (236 mL) delivers 366 milligrams of potassium, representing 8% of the DV.

- Approximately 3/4 cup (or 214 grams) of natural Greek yogurt contains 240 milligrams of potassium, contributing 5% to the DV.

- A medium-sized tomato (123 grams) contains 6% of the DV for sodium.

- A cup (235 mL) of brewed coffee provides 116 milligrams of caffeine, amounting to 2% of the DV.

While increasing potassium intake alone might not be the most effective strategy for addressing low potassium levels, it remains advisable for overall health. Fruits, vegetables, legumes, and dairy products are excellent sources of potassium owing to their wholesome nature. Presently, the recommended Adequate Intakes (AI) for men and women are 3,400 and 2,600 milligrams, respectively. Therefore, incorporating potassium-rich foods into your diet is essential for maintaining optimal health and well-being.

Avoiding Hypokalemia

Hypokalemia, a condition characterized by low levels of potassium in the body, is a prevalent concern among individuals undergoing hospitalization, affecting around 20% of patients in such settings. Conversely, its occurrence in the general population outside healthcare facilities is relatively rare, affecting only about 1% of individuals.

In the clinical setting, medical practitioners, including physicians and nurses, adhere to established protocols for monitoring patients' potassium levels to prevent hypokalemia during their hospital stays. This vigilance is crucial, given the potential complications associated with electrolyte imbalances.

The onset of severe symptoms such as prolonged nausea, vomiting, or diarrhea lasting beyond 24 to 48 hours warrants prompt medical attention. Preventing protracted periods of illness and fluid loss is paramount in mitigating the risk of hypokalemia and its adverse effects on health.

While hypokalemia is rarely attributed to a low-potassium diet, the significance of potassium in maintaining bodily functions cannot be overstated. Emphasizing the role of potassium-rich foods in supporting overall health is essential, although dietary modifications should be made under the guidance of a healthcare professional.

Incorporating potassium-rich foods into one's daily diet is advisable to lower the risk of hypokalemia. Consulting with a healthcare provider can yield personalized dietary recommendations tailored to individual needs. Examples of potassium-rich foods include avocados, bananas, various beans and peas, bran, dark leafy greens, fish, lean meats, dairy products, oranges, peanut butter, potatoes, spinach, and tomatoes.

Prompt medical intervention is crucial if symptoms of vomiting and diarrhea persist beyond 24 to 48 hours, as prolonged fluid loss can exacerbate hypokalemia. Timely medical attention enhances the prospects of avoiding complications and achieving a complete recovery.

CHAPTER IV: NUTRITIOUS LOW-POTASSIUM DISHES

BREAKFAST WITH LOW POTASSIUM

Sweet Coconut Oatmeal

Things Needed

1 (14 ounce) can coconut milk

1 cup rolled oats

2 tablespoons honey

¼ cup coconut flakes (Optional)

2 tablespoons brown sugar, or more to taste

1 teaspoon ground cinnamon

Preparation

Bring coconut milk to a gentle boil in a small saucepan over medium-low heat. Stir in oats and honey; lower heat and simmer until milk has mostly been absorbed, about 15 minutes.

Sprinkle coconut flakes, brown sugar, and cinnamon into oatmeal. Cook until oats are creamy and flavors are combined, about 5 minutes.

Scrambled Eggs and Tomatoes

Things Needed

2 large eggs, beaten

2 tomatoes, coarsely chopped

1 ½ teaspoons sugar

salt to taste

1 dash soy sauce

Preparation

In a skillet over medium heat, scramble eggs until almost done. Remove to a plate.

Return skillet to medium heat, and stir in tomatoes. Cook 2 to 3 minutes. Stir in sugar, salt, and soy. Return eggs to skillet; cook, stirring, about 1 minute more.

Potato Pancakes

Things Needed

5 medium potatoes, peeled and shredded

1 medium onion, finely chopped

2 large eggs, beaten

3 tablespoons all-purpose flour

salt and pepper to taste

3 tablespoons vegetable oil

Preparation

Combine potatoes, onion, eggs, flour, salt, and pepper in a large bowl; stir until well combined. Heat oil in a large skillet over medium-high heat. Working in batches, drop large spoonfuls of potato batter into the hot skillet. Flatten batter lightly with a spatula and cook until golden brown, about 4 minutes per side. Serve immediately.

Potato and Egg Frittata

Things Needed

2 tablespoons olive oil

1 large baking potato, peeled and sliced 1/4 inch thick

6 eggs, beaten

salt and pepper to taste

Preparation

Heat oil in a large skillet or frying pan over medium-high heat. Spread potato slices across bottom of the pan and cook, turning once, until golden on both sides. Remove slices from pan and drain.

When all potato slices have been cooked, return them to the pan. Turn heat to high. Pour on the beaten eggs and season with salt and pepper. Tilt the pan so that the eggs flow to the bottom of the pan. Turn heat to medium low. Cover pan with a plate and flip pan so that frittata is turned out onto plate. Slide the frittata back into the pan with the uncooked side down. Cover and let cook another 2 minutes.

When frittata is finished cooking, remove it from the pan and drain briefly on paper towels before serving.

Brown Rice Breakfast Porridge

Things Needed

1 cup cooked brown rice

1 cup 2% low-fat milk

2 tablespoons dried blueberries

1 dash cinnamon

1 tablespoon honey

1 egg

¼ teaspoon vanilla extract

1 tablespoon butter

Preparation

Combine the cooked brown rice, milk, blueberries, cinnamon, and honey in a small saucepan. Bring to a boil, then reduce heat to low and simmer for 20 minutes.

Beat the egg in a small bowl. Temper the egg by whisking in some of the hot rice, a tablespoon at a time until you have incorporated about 6 tablespoons. Stir the egg into the rice along with the vanilla and butter, and continue cooking over low heat for 1 to 2 minutes to thicken.

Fresh Sweet Corn Fritters

Things Needed

1 cup all-purpose flour

1 teaspoon baking powder

3 ears fresh corn, kernels cut from cob

2 eggs, separated

½ cup heavy whipping cream

salt and freshly ground pepper to taste

1 quart vegetable oil for frying, or as needed

2 tablespoons cane syrup, or as desired (Optional)

Preparation

Whisk flour and baking powder into a bowl and mix in corn kernels. Whisk egg yolks with cream in a small bowl and stir into the corn mixture; season with salt and black pepper. Beat egg whites with an electric mixer until fluffy and stiff peaks form in a separate bowl. Gently fold egg whites into the batter, retaining as much volume as possible.

Pour vegetable oil into a deep heavy skillet to a depth of 3 inches. Heat to 375 degrees F (190 degrees C).

Drop fritters into the hot oil, 2 to 3 tablespoons at a time, and cook until golden brown, 2 to 3 minutes per side. Drain fritters on paper towels and serve drizzled with cane syrup.

Mascarpone Stuffed French Toast with Peaches

Things Needed

8 fresh peaches

½ cup sugar

4 pinches ground nutmeg

½ teaspoon ground cinnamon

4 Mexican bolillo rolls

1 cup mascarpone cheese

6 tablespoons confectioners' sugar

1 lemon, zested

6 eggs

¾ cup milk

½ teaspoon vanilla extract

2 teaspoons butter, or as needed

2 teaspoons vegetable oil, or as needed

Preparation

Peel peaches, remove pits, and slice into a heavy saucepan, catching all the juices. Stir in sugar, nutmeg, and cinnamon, and cook over medium heat until bubbly. Continue cooking, stirring occasionally, until the sauce reaches a syrupy consistency, about 10 minutes. Remove from heat. Meanwhile, cut off and discard the ends of the bolillo rolls. Slice the rolls into 1 1/4-inch-thick slices. Lay each slice of bread on a board, and with a sharp knife held parallel to the board, cut a pocket into each slice, leaving three sides intact. Set aside.

Stir together the mascarpone, confectioners' sugar, and lemon zest until smooth. Scoop this mixture into a small plastic bag. Cut off one corner of the bag, and pipe as much filling into the pocket in each slice of bread as will fit without overflowing.

Whisk together the eggs, milk, and vanilla in a shallow bowl. Melt butter with oil over medium heat in a large nonstick skillet. Dip each stuffed piece of bread into the batter, add to the skillet, and cook until browned on both sides. Serve hot with the warm peach sauce.

Crab Omelet

Things Needed

2 tablespoons olive oil

1 small potato, peeled and diced

1 onion, chopped

2 cloves garlic, minced

¼ pound fresh crabmeat, drained and flaked

salt and pepper to taste

1 small tomato, diced

1 (1.5 ounce) box raisins

¼ cup peas

1 red bell pepper, chopped

3 eggs, beaten

Preparation

Heat olive oil in a skillet over medium heat. Fry potato in hot oil until fork-tender, 5 to 7 minutes.

Use a slotted spoon to transfer potatoes to a plate lined with paper towels, leaving excess oil in the skillet.

Return the skillet to medium heat. Cook onion and garlic in oil until tender, about 5 minutes. Add crab to the skillet and season with salt and pepper; stir. Cover the skillet and cook for 2 minutes. Stir tomatoes into mixture and cook another 2 minutes. Add raisins, peas, and red bell pepper; stir and cook another 2 minutes.

Pour eggs over mixture in the skillet. Cook until eggs set, 2 to 3 minutes. Flip omelet and cook 1 minute more. Transfer to a plate and serve hot with potatoes.

Roasted Butternut Squash Soufflé

Things Needed

1 tablespoon white sugar, or as needed

1 (2 pound) butternut squash, halved and seeded

¼ cup all-purpose flour

½ teaspoon baking powder

¼ teaspoon salt

½ cup unsalted butter at room temperature

¼ cup white sugar

¼ cup brown sugar

1 teaspoon vanilla extract

½ teaspoon ground cinnamon

¼ teaspoon ground nutmeg

3 large eggs at room temperature, separated

Preparation

Preheat the oven to 350 degrees F (175 degrees C). Line a baking sheet with parchment paper. Lightly butter a 2-quart soufflé or ceramic baking dish; sprinkle 1 tablespoon white sugar over butter, tapping excess sugar out of the dish. Store the prepared dish in the refrigerator.

Place butternut squash, cut-sides down, onto the prepared baking sheet.

Bake in the preheated oven until very soft, 1 to 1 1/2 hours. Allow squash to cool to room temperature.

Sift together flour, baking powder, and salt in a bowl; set aside.

Scrape flesh from butternut squash into a food processor and process until smooth. Add flour mixture, butter, 1/4 cup white sugar, brown sugar, vanilla, cinnamon, and nutmeg; process until smooth. Add egg yolks, one at a time, to squash mixture while continuously processing. Transfer squash mixture to a large bowl.

Beat egg whites in a bowl with an electric mixer until stiff peaks form; fold into squash mixture. Pour mixture into the chilled dish.

Bake in the preheated oven until the top is browned and springs back when gently pressed, about 1 hour.

Apple Cinnamon Oatmeal

Things Needed

1 cup water

¼ cup apple juice

1 apple, cored and chopped

⅔ cup rolled oats

1 teaspoon ground cinnamon

1 cup milk

Preparation

Combine the water, apple juice, and apples in a saucepan. Bring to a boil over high heat, and stir in the rolled oats and cinnamon. Return to a boil, then reduce heat to low, and simmer until thick, about 3 minutes. Spoon into serving bowls, and pour milk over the servings.

Egg Bites

Things Needed

cooking spray

5 small tri-color baby potatoes, thinly sliced

¼ stick butter

10 small eggs

1 small yellow bell pepper, finely chopped

1 small tomato, finely chopped

½ cup fresh spinach

¼ cup chopped ham

¼ cup chopped white onion

1 slice mozzarella cheese, cut into 12 cubes

Preparation

Preheat the oven to 350 degrees F (175 degrees C).

Spray a 12-cup muffin tin with nonstick cooking spray.

Place a thin layer of potato slices in the bottom of each muffin cup. Add a little butter on top.

Bake in the preheated oven for 5 minutes.

Mix together eggs, bell pepper, tomato, spinach, ham, and onion in a large bowl. Ladle egg mixture over warm potatoes. Top each muffin cup with a mozzarella cube.

Continue baking until eggs are set, about 20 minutes.

Fereni Starch Pudding

Things Needed

⅔ cup cornstarch

2 cups milk, divided

½ cup ground almonds

6 whole cardamom seeds

¼ cup white sugar, or to taste

1/4 teaspoon rosewater, or to taste

¼ cup blanched slivered almonds

Preparation

Dissolve cornstarch in 1 cup milk in a small bowl; set aside.

Combine remaining 1 cup milk, ground almonds, and cardamom in a medium pot; bring to a boil.

Reduce heat to medium and whisk in cornstarch mixture. Mix in sugar and rosewater. Allow pudding to boil, stirring constantly, for about 3 minutes.

Remove cardamom seeds and pour pudding into serving dishes. Garnish with slivered almonds and serve warm or cold.

Spanish Potato Omelet

Things Needed

½ cup olive oil

½ pound potatoes, thinly sliced

salt and pepper to taste

1 large onion, thinly sliced

4 large eggs

2 medium tomatoes - peeled, seeded, and coarsely chopped

2 green onions, chopped

Preparation

Heat oil over medium-high heat in a large skillet. Add potatoes and season lightly with salt and pepper; cook, stirring occasionally, until golden brown and crisp, 10 to 14 minutes. Add onions; cook and stir until soft and beginning to brown, 6 to 8 minutes.

Whisk eggs in a bowl; season with salt and pepper. Pour eggs into the skillet and stir gently to combine with potatoes and onion. Reduce the heat to low and cook until eggs begin to brown on the bottom, 4 to 5 minutes.

Loosen omelet with a spatula. Invert a large plate over the pan, and carefully flip omelet out onto the plate. Slide omelet, uncooked-side down, back into the pan. Cook until eggs are set, 4 to 5 minutes. Serve warm, garnished with tomato and green onion.

Bionicos (Mexican Fruit Bowls)

Things Needed

Topping:

⅓ cup plain yogurt

⅓ cup sweetened condensed milk

⅓ cup Mexican crema

1 teaspoon vanilla extract

Fruit Salad:

1 cup diced cantaloupe

1 cup diced papaya

1 cup diced red apple

1 cup sliced banana

1 cup sliced strawberries

½ cup granola

½ cup raisins

½ cup shredded coconut

Preparation

Make the topping: Mix yogurt, condensed milk, Mexican crema, and vanilla together in a bowl until well combined.

Make the fruit salads: Divide cantaloupe, papaya, apple, and banana among 4 individual bowls, arranging each fruit in its own section. Place strawberries in the center of each bowl. Sprinkle granola, raisins, and coconut over the bowls, then drizzle with the topping.

Pierogi Dough

Things Needed

4 cups all-purpose flour

1 teaspoon salt

2 teaspoons vegetable oil

¼ teaspoon baking powder

1 cup warm water

1 egg, beaten

Preparation

In a large bowl mix together the flour, salt, and baking powder. Make a well in the center.

In a separate bowl mix together the vegetable oil, warm water, and beaten egg. Pour into the well of the dry Things Needed. Knead dough for 8 to 10 minutes.

Cover dough and let rest for 2 hours. Roll out and fill as desired.

LOW POTASSIUM LUNCH RECIPES

Roast Chicken with Rosemary

Things Needed

1 (3 pound) whole chicken, rinsed

salt and pepper to taste

1 small onion, quartered

¼ cup chopped fresh rosemary

Preparation

Preheat the oven to 350 degrees F (175 degrees C). Season chicken all over with salt and pepper, including cavity. Stuff cavity with onion and rosemary. Place chicken in a 9x13-inch baking dish or roasting pan.

Roast in the preheated oven until chicken is no longer pink in the center and the juices run clear, 2 to 2 1/2 hours. An instant-read thermometer inserted into the center of chicken near the bone should read at least 165 degrees F (74 degrees C).

Traditional Gyro Meat

Things Needed

½ onion, cut into chunks

1 pound ground lamb

1 pound ground beef

1 tablespoon minced garlic

1 teaspoon dried oregano

1 teaspoon ground cumin

1 teaspoon dried marjoram

1 teaspoon ground dried rosemary

1 teaspoon ground dried thyme

1 teaspoon ground black pepper

¼ teaspoon sea salt

Preparation

Pulse onion in a food processor until finely chopped. Scoop onions onto the center of a towel, gather up the towel ends, and squeeze to remove liquid.

Combine onions, lamb, beef, garlic, oregano, cumin, marjoram, rosemary, thyme, pepper, and salt in a large bowl. Mix with your hands until well combined. Cover and refrigerate 1 to 2 hours to allow the flavors to blend.

Preheat the oven to 325 degrees F (165 degrees C).

Place the meat mixture into a food processor and pulse until finely chopped and the texture feels tacky, about 1 minute. Transfer to a 7x4-inch loaf pan, and pack down to make sure there are no air pockets.

Line a large roasting pan with a damp kitchen towel. Place the loaf pan in the center of the towel-lined roasting pan, and transfer it into the preheated oven. Carefully pour boiling water into the roasting pan until it comes halfway up the sides of the loaf pan.

Bake in the preheated oven until gyro meat is no longer pink in the center, about 45 minutes to 1 hour. An instant-read thermometer inserted into the center should read at least 160 degrees F (70 degrees C).

Pour off any accumulated fat, and allow to cool slightly before slicing thinly and serving.

Southern Fried Chicken Livers

Things Needed

1 pound chicken livers

1 egg

½ cup milk

1 cup all-purpose flour

1 tablespoon garlic powder

salt and pepper to taste

1 quart vegetable oil for frying

Preparation

Place chicken livers in a colander; rinse with cold water and drain well. Blot dry with paper towels. Whisk egg and milk together in a shallow dish until blended.

Place flour, garlic powder, salt, and pepper into a zip-top bag; shake to combine.

Heat oil in a deep fryer or large saucepan to 375 degrees F (190 degrees C).

Dip chicken livers in egg mixture to coat, then transfer, one at a time, into flour mixture, shaking the bag to coat completely.

Gently place coated livers, a few at a time, into hot oil; cover with a splatter screen and cook until crisp and golden brown, 5 to 6 minutes.

Pinakbet

Things Needed

3 tablespoons olive oil

1 onion, chopped

2 cloves garlic, minced

½ pound pork loin, chopped

½ pound peeled and deveined prawns

salt and pepper to taste

1 tomato, chopped

¼ pound zucchini, seeded and cut into bite-size pieces

¼ pound fresh okra, ends trimmed

¼ pound fresh green beans, trimmed

¼ pound eggplant, cut into bite-size pieces

1 small bitter melon, cut into bite-size pieces

Preparation

Heat oil in a large pot over medium heat; stir in onion and garlic and cook until tender, about 5 minutes.

Add pork; cook and stir until browned, 5 to 7 minutes.

Add prawns; cook and stir until they turn pink, about 5 minutes.

Stir in tomato; season with salt and pepper, cover and simmer for 5 minutes.

Stir in zucchini, okra, green beans, eggplant, and bitter melon; cover and cook until the vegetables are tender, about 10 minutes.

Tri Tip Roast

Things Needed

1 (1 1/2 pound) beef tri tip roast, trimmed

1 teaspoon dried thyme

1 teaspoon dried basil

1 teaspoon dried marjoram

1 teaspoon dry mustard

salt and ground black pepper to taste

⅓ cup red wine

1 tablespoon olive oil, or as needed

Preparation

Rub beef all over with thyme, basil, marjoram, dry mustard, salt, and black pepper; transfer into a re-sealable plastic bag. Seal the bag and refrigerate, 8 hours to overnight. Pour red wine into the bag 4 hours before cooking.

Preheat the oven to 450 degrees F (230 degrees C). Drizzle olive oil over the bottom of a roasting pan; transfer beef into the prepared roasting pan.

Roast in the preheated oven for 15 minutes. Reduce oven temperature to 350 degrees F (175 degrees C) and continue roasting until slightly pink in the center, 20 to 25 minutes more. An instant-read thermometer inserted into the center should read 140 degrees F (60 degrees C).

Let rest for 5 to 10 minutes before thinly slicing against the grain.

Spicy Tuna Rolls

Things Needed

4 sheets nori (dry seaweed)

½ pound sashimi-grade tuna, finely chopped

4 tablespoons mayonnaise

2 green onions, chopped

1 tablespoon hot chile sauce

2 ½ cups prepared sushi rice

1 tablespoon sesame seeds

Preparation

Cut off the bottom quarter of each nori sheet; reserve for another use.

Combine chopped tuna, mayonnaise, green onions, and hot sauce in a bowl.

Center 1 sheet of nori on a bamboo sushi mat. Wet your hands. Spread a thin layer of rice on the nori using your hands; press into a thin layer, leaving a 1/2-inch space at the bottom edge.

Sprinkle with sesame seeds. Arrange 1/4 of the tuna mixture in a line across the rice, about 1/3 of the way down from the top of the sheet.

Wet the uncovered edge of the nori. Lift the top end of the mat and firmly roll it over the Things Needed. Roll it forward to make a complete roll. Repeat with remaining Things Needed.

Slice the rolls into 3/4-inch pieces using a wet knife. Serve immediately or refrigerate until serving.

Penne with Chicken and Asparagus

Things Needed

1 (16 ounce) package dried penne pasta

5 tablespoons olive oil, divided

2 skinless, boneless chicken breast halves - cut into cubes

¼ teaspoon garlic powder, or more to taste

salt and ground black pepper to taste

½ cup low-sodium chicken broth

1 bunch slender asparagus spears, trimmed, cut on diagonal into 1-inch pieces

1 clove garlic, thinly sliced

¼ cup grated Parmesan cheese

Preparation

Bring a large pot of lightly salted water to a boil. Add penne and cook, stirring occasionally, until tender yet firm to the bite, about 11 minutes. Drain. While the pasta is cooking, heat 3 tablespoons oil in a large skillet over medium-high heat. Stir in chicken and season with 1/4 teaspoon garlic powder, salt, and pepper. Cook and stir until chicken is browned and the juices run clear, about 5 minutes. Transfer chicken to a paper towel-lined plate.

Pour chicken broth into the skillet. Add asparagus, garlic, and another pinch of garlic powder. Season with salt and pepper. Cover and steam until asparagus is just tender, 5 to 10 minutes. Return chicken to the skillet and cook until heated through, 2 to 3 minutes.

Transfer drained penne to a large bowl. Pour chicken mixture over top and mix until well combined. Let sit for about 5 minutes.

Stir in remaining 2 tablespoons olive oil, then sprinkle with Parmesan cheese.

Turkey Kofta Kebabs

Things Needed

vegetable oil for grill

1 pound ground turkey

1 small onion, minced

¼ cup chopped fresh cilantro

1 large egg

2 cloves garlic, minced

¼ teaspoon chopped green chile pepper

¼ teaspoon ground coriander

¼ teaspoon ground paprika

¼ teaspoon chili powder

salt to taste

Preparation

Preheat the grill for medium heat and lightly oil the grate.

Combine turkey, onion, cilantro, egg, garlic, chile pepper, coriander, paprika, chili powder, and salt in a large bowl; mix thoroughly. Divide mixture into twelve 1/4-cup portions; roll into log-shaped ovals and place on a baking sheet.

Grill ovals over indirect heat, turning occasionally, until no longer pink in the center, 25 to 30 minutes. An instant-read thermometer inserted into the center should read at least 165 degrees F (74 degrees C).

Lamb Chops with Balsamic Reduction

Things Needed

¾ teaspoon dried rosemary

½ teaspoon dried thyme

¼ teaspoon dried basil

salt and pepper to taste

4 lamb chops (3/4 inch thick)

1 tablespoon olive oil

¼ cup minced shallots

⅓ cup aged balsamic vinegar

¾ cup chicken broth

1 tablespoon butter

Preparation

Gather all Things Needed.

Mix rosemary, thyme, basil, salt, and pepper together in a small bowl; rub onto chops, coating both sides. Place chops onto a plate, cover, and let sit for 15 minutes.

Heat oil in a large skillet over medium-high heat. Cook chops in the hot skillet until no longer pink in the center, about 3 1/2 minutes per side for medium-rare. An instant-read thermometer inserted into the center should read 145 degrees F (63 degrees C). Transfer to a serving platter and keep warm.

Add shallots to the skillet; cook and stir until just browned, 2 to 3 minutes. Pour vinegar into the pan and bring to a boil while scraping the browned bits of food off the bottom of the pan with a wooden spoon. Add broth; cook and stir until sauce has reduced by half, about 5 minutes.

Remove sauce from the heat and stir in butter until melted.

Serve over chops. Enjoy!

Filipino Lumpia

Things Needed

1 (12 ounce) package lumpia wrappers

1 pound ground beef

½ pound ground pork

⅓ cup finely chopped onion

⅓ cup finely chopped green bell pepper

⅓ cup finely chopped carrot

1 quart oil for frying

Preparation

Make sure the lumpia wrappers are completely thawed. Lay several out on a clean dry surface and cover with a damp towel. The wrappers are very thin and the edges will dry out quickly.

In a medium bowl, blend together the ground beef and pork, onion, green pepper and carrot. Place about 2 tablespoons of the meat mixture along the center of the wrapper. The filling should be no bigger around than your thumb or the wrapper will burn before the meat is cooked. Fold one edge of the wrapper over to the other. Fold the outer edges in slightly, then continue to roll into a cylinder. Wet your finger, and moisten the edge to seal. Repeat with the remaining wrappers and filling, keeping finished lumpias covered to prevent drying. This is a good time to recruit a friend or loved one to make the job less repetitive!! Heat oil in a 9 inch skillet at medium to medium high heat until oil is 365 to 375 degrees F (170 to 175 degrees C) Fry 3-4 lumpia at a time. It should only take about 2-3 minutes for each side. The lumpia will be nicely browned when done. Drain on paper towels.

You can cut each lumpia into thirds for parties, if you like.

High Temperature Eye-of-Round Roast

Things Needed

1 (3 pound) beef eye of round roast

salt and pepper to taste

Preparation

Preheat the oven to 500 degrees F (260 degrees C).

Season roast with salt and pepper; place in a roasting pan or baking dish. Do not cover or add water.

Place roast in the preheated oven and reduce temperature to 475 degrees F (245 degrees C). Roast for 21 minutes (7 minutes per pound), then turn off the oven and let roast sit in the hot oven for 2 1/2 hours. Do not open the door at all during this time.

Remove roast from the oven and check that the internal temperature is at least 145 degrees F (65 degrees C). Carve into thin slices to serve.

Baked Salmon in Foil

Things Needed

½ cup olive oil

5 cloves cloves garlic, minced or pressed through a garlic press

2 ½ tablespoons fresh lemon juice, or more to taste

1 tablespoon brown sugar

1 teaspoon dried oregano

1 teaspoon dried thyme

salt and freshly ground black pepper to taste

aluminum foil

1 teaspoon olive oil

1 (3 pound) salmon fillet

¼ cup chopped fresh parsley

1 lemon, sliced

Preparation

Preheat the oven to 375 degrees F (190 degrees C).
Combine 1/2 cup olive oil, garlic, lemon juice,
brown sugar, oregano, thyme, salt, and pepper in
a bowl.

Place a large piece of aluminum foil on a baking
sheet and brush with 1 teaspoon olive oil. Place

salmon, skin-side down, in the middle of the foil. Drizzle with olive oil mixture.

Fold up the edges of the foil over salmon to create a packet, making sure to seal the edges.

Bake in the preheated oven until fish flakes easily with a fork, 20 to 25 minutes. Garnish with fresh parsley and lemon slices.

Lemon Garlic Tilapia

Things Needed

nonstick cooking spray

4 tilapia fillets

3 tablespoons fresh lemon juice

1 tablespoon butter, melted

1 clove garlic, finely chopped

1 teaspoon dried parsley flakes

1 dash pepper to taste

Preparation

Preheat the oven to 375 degrees F (190 degrees C).

Spray a baking dish with nonstick cooking spray.

Rinse tilapia fillets under cool water, and pat dry with paper towels.

Place fillets in the prepared baking dish. Pour lemon juice over fillets, then drizzle butter on top.

Sprinkle with garlic, parsley, and pepper.

Bake in the preheated oven until fish is white and flakes when pulled apart with a fork, about 30 minutes.

Tofu Burgers

Things Needed

1 (12 ounce) package firm tofu, frozen for 72 hours

2 teaspoons vegetable oil

1 small onion, chopped

1 stalk celery, chopped

¼ cup shredded Cheddar cheese

1 large egg, beaten

salt and pepper to taste

½ cup vegetable oil for frying, or as needed

Preparation

Bring a large saucepan of water to a simmer. Leave frozen tofu in its package and place into the water. Remove from the heat and let tofu thaw for about 20 minutes in the hot water.

Remove tofu from the package and transfer to a plate. Place another plate on top of tofu. Set a 3- to 5-pound weight on top. Press tofu for 20 to 30 minutes; drain and discard the accumulated liquid.

While tofu is draining, heat 2 teaspoons oil in a small skillet over medium heat. Add onion and celery; sauté until soft and lightly browned, about 5 minutes. Remove from the heat.

Finely chop tofu and place into a mixing bowl. Add onion and celery mixture, Cheddar, egg, salt, and pepper; mix until thoroughly combined.

Pour 1/4 inch oil into a large skillet and heat over medium-high heat. Drop tofu mixture into the skillet in six equal portions. Flatten with a spatula to form patties. Fry until golden brown, 5 to 7 minutes per side.

Garlic Shrimp Kabobs

Things Needed

1 pound frozen shrimp, thawed and peeled

¼ cup olive oil

1 tablespoon minced garlic

2 teaspoons lemon juice

¼ teaspoon pepper

1 pinch finely chopped parsley

metal skewers

cooking spray

Preparation

Rinse and dry shrimp.

Whisk olive oil, garlic, lemon juice, pepper, and parsley together in a bowl and pour into a large resealable plastic bag. Add shrimp, coat with the marinade, squeeze out excess air, and seal the bag. Marinate in the refrigerator for 2 hours.

Preheat an outdoor grill for medium heat and lightly oil the grate. Lightly coat metal skewers with cooking spray.

Remove shrimp from the marinade and shake off excess. Discard the remaining marinade. Place about 5 shrimp on each skewer.

Cook on the preheated grill until shrimp are bright pink on the outside and the meat is opaque, about 5 minutes; do not overcook.

DINNER WITH MINIMAL POTASSIUM

Peruvian Causa

Things Needed

8 russet potatoes, peeled

½ cup vegetable oil, or as needed

2 tablespoons minced aji amarillo

salt and ground black pepper to taste

2 (5 ounce) cans tuna, drained

1 small red onion, diced small

½ cup mayonnaise, divided

2 avocados, cut into thin strips

3 hard-boiled eggs, thinly sliced

Preparation

Place potatoes into a large pot and cover with salted water; bring to a boil. Reduce heat to medium-low and simmer until tender, about 20 minutes. Drain.

Mash potatoes with a ricer or hand mixer until smooth. Gradually stir in oil until potatoes come together; add aji amarillo, salt, and pepper. Cool potato mixture in the refrigerator, about 20 minutes.

Stir tuna, onion, and 1/4 cup mayonnaise together in a bowl.

Line a casserole dish with plastic wrap. Spread 1/2 the potato mixture on the bottom of the dish. Spread 2 tablespoons mayonnaise over potatoes, spread tuna mixture over mayonnaise, and place avocado slices in a single layer on top of tuna mixture. Spread remaining 1/2 of potato mixture over avocados, and top with remaining 2 tablespoons mayonnaise. Place sliced eggs over top. Cover casserole dish with plastic wrap and refrigerate until firm, about 30 minutes.

Invert casserole dish onto a serving dish or baking sheet to remove potato casserole from dish. Remove plastic wrap and cut casserole into squares.

Easy Pan-Fried Fish Fillet

Things Needed

4 (5 ounce) mild white fish fillets

1 lemon, juiced

salt to taste

4 tablespoons all-purpose flour

1 teaspoon five-spice powder

4 tablespoons canola oil

1 tablespoon sesame oil (Optional)

Preparation

Wash fish under cold running water, then pat dry with paper towels. Drizzle with lemon juice and season with salt on both sides.

Combine flour and five-spice powder in a shallow bowl. Dip fish fillets into flour mixture to coat on both sides.

Heat canola and sesame oils in a large skillet over medium heat. Add fish and pan-fry for 2 to 3 minutes. Use two spatulas to carefully flip fillets; continue cooking until fish flakes easily with a fork, 2 to 3 more minutes.

Easy Lemon Pepper Blackened Salmon

Things Needed

2 tablespoons butter, melted

2 tablespoons fresh lemon juice

1 teaspoon chopped fresh parsley

½ teaspoon garlic powder

salt and ground black pepper to taste

1 tablespoon whole black peppercorns

4 salmon fillets

2 tablespoons olive oil

Preparation

Preheat the oven to 350 degrees F (175 degrees C).

Whisk together butter, lemon juice, parsley, garlic

powder, salt, and pepper in a medium bowl. Stir

in peppercorns. Dip salmon fillets, one at a time,

into lemon mixture so the flesh side is coated. Place coated fillets onto a plate.

Heat olive oil in a large, oven-proof skillet over medium-high heat. Once oil begins to smoke, place salmon, skin-side up, into the skillet. Cook in hot oil until flesh is seared and golden brown, about 1 minute.

Place the skillet into the preheated oven and cook until salmon flakes easily with a fork, 10 to 12 minutes.

Citrus Swordfish with Citrus Salsa

Things Needed

Salsa:

1 medium orange, peeled, sectioned, and cut into bite-size

½ cup canned pineapple chunks, undrained

¼ cup diced fresh mango

2 medium jalapeno peppers, seeded and minced

3 tablespoons orange juice

1 tablespoon diced red bell pepper

2 teaspoons white sugar

1 tablespoon chopped fresh cilantro

Swordfish:

½ cup fresh orange juice

1 tablespoon olive oil

1 tablespoon pineapple juice concentrate, thawed

¼ teaspoon cayenne pepper

1 ½ pounds swordfish steaks

Preparation

Make the salsa: Mix orange, pineapple, mango, jalapeños, orange juice, bell pepper, sugar, and cilantro together in a medium bowl until well combined. Cover and refrigerate until needed.

Marinate the swordfish: Whisk orange juice, oil, pineapple juice concentrate, and cayenne together in a large glass or ceramic bowl. Add swordfish and turn to evenly coat. Cover the bowl with plastic wrap and marinate in the refrigerator for 30 minutes.

Preheat an outdoor grill for medium-high heat and lightly oil the grate.

Remove swordfish from marinade and shake off excess. Discard remaining marinade.

Grill on the preheated grill until opaque in the center, 6 to 8 minutes per side. Serve with the salsa.

Shrimp and Sugar Snap Peas

Things Needed

1 (16 ounce) package uncooked linguini pasta

2 tablespoons olive oil

1 teaspoon chili oil

1 ½ pounds medium shrimp, peeled and deveined

1 pound sugar snap pea pods

2 large cloves garlic, minced

1 ½ cups dry white wine

¼ cup reserved pasta water

1 tablespoon unsalted butter

1 tablespoon fresh lemon juice

⅓ cup chopped fresh basil

Preparation

Bring a large pot of lightly salted water to a boil. Add linguini pasta, and cook for 8 to 10 minutes or until al dente. Drain, reserving 1/4 cup liquid.

Heat the olive oil and chili oil in a wok over medium-high heat. Mix in the shrimp, pea pods, and garlic. Cook and stir 2 minutes, until shrimp are almost opaque. Remove from heat, and set aside.

Pour the wine into the wok, and bring to a boil. Cook until reduced by 1/3. Return shrimp, peas, and garlic to the wok, and stir in the reserved pasta water. Continue to cook and stir until shrimp are opaque. Remove wok from heat, and mix in the butter, lemon juice, and basil. Toss with the cooked pasta to serve.

Lime-Marinated Mahi Mahi

Things Needed

¾ cup extra-virgin olive oil

2 tablespoons lime juice

1 clove garlic, minced

½ teaspoon cayenne pepper

⅛ teaspoon grated lime zest (Optional)

⅛ teaspoon ground black pepper

1 pinch salt

2 (4 ounce) mahi mahi fillets

2 twists lime zest (Optional)

Preparation

Whisk olive oil, lime juice, garlic, cayenne pepper, lime zest, black pepper, and salt together in a bowl. Add mahi mahi fillets and turn to coat. Let marinate for at least 15 minutes.

Preheat an outdoor grill for medium heat and lightly oil the grate.

Remove mahi mahi from marinade and shake off excess. Discard remaining marinade.

Cook mahi mahi on the preheated grill until fish flakes easily with a fork and is lightly browned, 3 to 4 minutes per side. Garnish with the twists of lime zest to serve.

Broiled Spanish Mackerel

Things Needed

6 (3 ounce) fillets Spanish mackerel fillets

¼ cup olive oil

½ teaspoon paprika

salt and ground black pepper to taste

12 slices lemon

Preparation

Preheat the oven's broiler and set the oven rack about 6 inches from the heat source. Lightly grease a baking dish.

Rub both sides of each mackerel fillet with olive oil and place with the skin side down into the prepared baking dish. Season each fillet with the paprika, salt, and pepper. Top each fillet with two lemon slices.

Bake the fillets under the broiler until the fish just begins to flake, 5 to 7 minutes. Serve immediately.

Fried Soft-Shell Crab

Things Needed

4 soft-shell crabs

1 quart oil for frying, or as needed

½ cup milk

1 large egg

1 cup all-purpose flour

salt and pepper to taste

Preparation

Lift one pointed side of the top shell of one crab; pull out and discard the gills. Lower the shell and repeat on the other side. Remove the tail flap on the bottom side by twisting and pulling. Use a pair of scissors to cut behind the eyes and remove the face. Repeat to clean remaining crabs. Rinse cleaned crabs thoroughly with cold water, then dry on paper towels.

Heat oil in a deep fryer to 365 degrees F (180 degrees C).

Whisk together milk and egg in a shallow bowl. Combine flour, salt, and pepper in another shallow bowl. Lightly salt each crab. Dredge in flour; shake off excess. Dip into beaten egg. Lift up so excess egg drips back into the bowl. Press into flour to coat both sides.

Working in batches if necessary, carefully lower crabs into the hot oil and fry until golden brown on one side, 1 to 2 minutes. Carefully turn and cook until golden brown on the other side, 1 to 2 minutes more. Drain on paper towels.

Pan-Seared Red Snapper

Things Needed

¼ cup chopped green onions

1 lemon, juiced

2 tablespoons rice wine vinegar

1 tablespoon olive oil

1 tablespoon honey

1 teaspoon Dijon mustard

1 teaspoon ground ginger

2 (4 ounce) fillets red snapper

Preparation

Gather all Things Needed.

Mix together green onions, lemon juice, vinegar, olive oil, honey, mustard, and ginger in a shallow bowl; set aside.

Rinse snapper under cold water and pat dry with paper towels.

Heat a large nonstick skillet over medium heat.

Dip snapper into marinade to coat both sides.

Cook snapper in the hot skillet until opaque and lightly browned, 2 to 3 minutes per side.

Pour remaining marinade into the skillet. Reduce heat and simmer until fish flakes easily with a fork, 2 to 3 minutes.

Clams and Garlic

Things Needed

50 small clams in shell, scrubbed

2 tablespoons extra virgin olive oil

6 cloves garlic, minced

1 cup white wine

2 tablespoons butter

½ cup chopped fresh parsley

Preparation

Gather all Things Needed.

Wash clams to remove any dirt or sand.

Heat oil in a large pot over medium heat. Sauté garlic in hot oil until tender, about 1 minute.

Pour in white wine; bring to a boil. Cook until wine is reduced by half.

Add clams, cover the pot, and steam just until clams start to open. Add butter, cover the pot, and continue cooking until most or all of the clams open. Discard any clams that do not open.

Transfer clams and broth to 2 large bowls. Sprinkle with chopped parsley and serve.

Stir-fried beef with hoisin sauce

Things Needed

1 tablespoon soy sauce

1 tablespoon dry sherry

2 tablespoon sesame oil

1 fat garlic clove, crushed

1 tablespoon finely chopped fresh root ginger (or fresh ginger paste in a jar)

200g lean sirloin steak, thinly sliced across the grain

1 tablespoon sesame seeds

1 tablespoon sunflower oil

1 large carrot, cut into matchsticks

100g mangetout, halved lengthways

140g mushrooms, sliced

3 tablespoon hoisin sauce

Chinese noodles, to serve

Preparation

Mix together the soy sauce, sherry, sesame oil, garlic and ginger in a shallow dish. Add the steak and leave to marinate for about 20 minutes (or longer, if you have time).

Heat a large heavy-based frying pan or wok, add the sesame seeds and toast over a high heat, stirring, for a few minutes until golden. Tip on to a plate.

When ready to cook, heat the sunflower oil in a large frying pan or wok until hot. Add the steak with the marinade and stir fry for 3-4 minutes over a high heat until lightly browned. Remove, using a slotted spoon, on to a plate, leaving the juices in the pan.

Toss the carrots in the pan and stir fry for a few minutes, then add the mangetout and cook for a further 2 minutes.

Return the steak to the pan, add the mushrooms and toss everything together. Add the hoisin sauce and stir fry for a final minute. Sprinkle with the toasted sesame seeds and serve immediately.

Ravioli with walnuts, goat's cheese & cavolo nero sauce

Things Needed

For the sauce

200g cavolo nero

75ml olive oil, plus extra to toss the pasta

1small garlic clove

1 lemon, juiced

8-12 fresh or dried lasagne sheets, depending on size

finely grated pecorino, parmesan or vegetarian alternative, to serve

For the goat's cheese paste

140g walnuts

handful sage leaves, chopped

120g goat's cheese

lemon juice, to taste

50ml olive oil

Preparation

Bring a large pan of lightly salted water to the boil, then add the cavolo nero. Cook for 1-2 minutes until the kale turns bright green and softens. Lift out with tongs into a colander, keeping the cooking water to boil the pasta. Run cold water over the kale, squeeze out any excess water, then transfer to a food processor. Add the oil, garlic, lemon juice and 1 tablespoon salt, then blitz to a fine pesto. Season to taste and transfer to a small pan. Gently warm over a medium-low heat.

Clean the food processor. For the goat's cheese paste, tip in the nuts, sage, goat's cheese, a good squeeze of lemon juice and the oil, then blitz to a paste. Season, then warm in another small pan over a medium-low heat, stirring occasionally.

Bring the pan of cavolo water to the boil again, adding more water if needed. Add the pasta sheets and simmer following pack instructions. Drain, keeping back a cup of the pasta water to add to the sauce (about 400ml). Cut the pasta sheets in half and toss in a little olive oil.

Stir the reserved pasta water through the cavolo sauce and keep on a low heat. If the sauce looks thick, thin down with a little more water, or increase the heat a little if too thin; it should be pourable like double cream. Spoon a pool of sauce onto each plate. Layer the lasagne sheets on top with spoonfuls of the goat's cheese paste in-between each layer. Top with the last sheet of pasta and ladle over a little more sauce, then scatter over the cheese.

Stuffed peppers with rice

Things Needed

4 red peppers

2 pouches cooked tomato rice

2 tablespoon pesto

handful pitted black olives, chopped

200g goat's cheese, sliced

Preparation

Use a small knife to cut the top out of 4 red peppers, then scoop out the seeds. Sit the peppers on a plate, cut-side up, and cook in the microwave on high for 5-6 minutes until they have wilted and softened.

While the peppers are cooking, mix two 250g pouches cooked tomato rice together with 2 tablespoon pesto and a handful of chopped pitted black olives and 140g of the sliced goat's cheese. Scoop the rice, pesto, olives and goat's cheese mix into the peppers, top with the remaining 60g sliced goat's cheese and continue to cook for 8-10 minutes.

Roasted Broccoli

Things Needed

14 ounces broccoli

1 tablespoon olive oil

salt and ground black pepper to taste

Preparation

Preheat the oven to 400 degrees F (200 degrees C).

Cut broccoli florets from the stalk. Peel the stalk and slice into 1/4-inch slices. Mix florets and stem pieces with olive oil in a bowl and transfer to a baking sheet; season with salt and pepper.

Roast in the preheated oven until broccoli is tender and lightly browned, about 18 to 20 minutes.

Oven-Baked Potato Slices

Things Needed

4 medium baking potatoes, sliced 1/8-inch thick

⅛ teaspoon garlic powder

⅛ teaspoon ground black pepper

⅛ teaspoon celery seed

⅛ teaspoon paprika

1 pinch cayenne pepper

1 dash salt

4 tablespoons olive oil, or more as needed

Preparation

Preheat the oven to 400 degrees F (200 degrees C).

Place potatoes, garlic powder, black pepper, celery seed, paprika, cayenne pepper, and salt into a zip-top bag. Shake to coat evenly.

Pour the entire contents of the bag onto a large baking sheet and spread evenly. Drizzle with olive oil.

Bake in the preheated oven until potatoes reach desired crispness, turning frequently to brown evenly, 40 to 45 minutes.

Remove from the oven. Let cool slightly and transfer into a serving dish.

LOW POTASSUIM SOUPS

Roasted Broccoli Soup

Things Needed

5 cups chopped broccoli florets and stalks

1 onion, chopped into 1-inch pieces

3 cloves garlic, peeled

2 tablespoons olive oil

3 cups vegetable broth

4 ounces cream cheese, softened

¾ teaspoon lemon pepper, or more as needed

crushed red pepper flakes to taste

Preparation

Preheat the oven to 400 degrees F (200 degrees C).

Line a baking sheet with parchment paper.

Place broccoli, onion, garlic, and olive oil in a large bowl and toss to coat evenly. Place on the prepared baking sheet in a single layer.

Roast vegetables until soft, 30 to 35 minutes, stirring every 10 minutes. Remove from oven. Chop 1/4 cup of broccoli florets; set aside for garnish.

Combine remaining vegetables with vegetable broth, cream cheese, and lemon pepper in a high-powered blender or food processor in batches. Puree soup until smooth.

Pour soup into a saucepan over medium-low heat until warmed through, about 5 minutes. Season with additional lemon pepper to taste. Ladle into bowls. Garnish with reserved chopped broccoli and crushed red pepper.

Watermelon Tomato Gazpacho with a Cool Cucumber Swirl

Things Needed

3 cups coarsely chopped seedless watermelon

¼ cup finely diced seedless watermelon

3 large Roma tomatoes, halved and seeded

1 small red bell pepper, roughly chopped

4 green onions, sliced, white parts and tops separated

3 tablespoons lemon juice

1 ½ teaspoons lime zest

2 tablespoons lime juice

1 tablespoon chopped fresh mint

1 tablespoon honey

⅛ teaspoon crushed red pepper, or to taste

1 large cucumber, peeled and seeded

1 clove garlic, minced

2 tablespoons chopped fresh parsley

⅓ cup vegetable broth

¼ cup sour cream

¼ teaspoon salt

¼ teaspoon ground black pepper

Preparation

For watermelon gazpacho, in a blender or food processor add coarsely chopped watermelon, 2 tomatoes, the bell pepper, the whites of green onions, 2 tablespoons lemon juice, 1 teaspoon lime zest, the lime juice, mint, honey, and crushed red pepper. Cover and blend or process until nearly smooth. Transfer to a large bowl. Chill, covered, 2 to 4 hours. Rinse blender or food processor.

For cucumber soup, finely chop 1/4 of the cucumber and coarsely chop remaining portion. Add coarsely chopped cucumber, garlic, parsley, green onion tops, and remaining lemon juice to blender or food processor. Cover and blend or process until nearly smooth. Transfer to large bowl. Stir in broth, sour cream, salt, and pepper. Chill, covered, 2 to 4 hours.

For tomato topper, chop remaining tomato into 1/2-inch pieces and add to small bowl. Stir in reserved finely chopped watermelon, finely chopped cucumber, and remaining lime zest. Chill, covered, until ready to serve.

To serve, ladle about 1 cup watermelon gazpacho into each bowl. Top each serving with about 1/2 cup cucumber soup and swirl slightly. Top with tomato topper and , if you like, additional black pepper and mint.

Butternut Bisque with French Onion Toast Topper

Things Needed

3 tablespoons butter

1 ½ cups chopped onion

1 ½ teaspoons kosher salt

2 tablespoons tomato paste

1 (2 pound) butternut squash - peeled, seeded, and cut into 1-inch cubes

4 cups low-sodium chicken broth

1 pinch cayenne pepper

½ cup heavy cream

2 tablespoons pure maple syrup

1 tablespoon chopped fresh parsley, or to taste

French Onion Toast Toppers:

3 tablespoons butter

1 tablespoon olive oil

3 large sweet onions, chopped

1 large shallot, thinly sliced

½ teaspoon salt

¼ teaspoon ground black pepper

2 tablespoons sherry

½ cup low-sodium beef broth

2 fresh thyme sprigs

6 slices sourdough bread

6 teaspoons butter, softened

6 ounces shredded Gruyere cheese

Preparation

Melt butter in a large pot over medium-low heat. Add onion and 1/2 teaspoon kosher salt. Cook, stirring frequently, until onion is tender but not browned, about 10 minutes.

Increase heat to medium-high. Stir in tomato paste. Cook, stirring frequently, until mixture begins to caramelize and brown, about 2 minutes. Add squash, chicken broth, remaining kosher salt, and cayenne pepper. Reduce heat to medium-low and simmer until squash is very tender, 20 to 25 minutes. Reduce heat to low.

Using an immersion blender, blend squash mixture until smooth. (Or transfer mixture, in batches if needed, to a blender or food processor. Cover and blend or process until smooth. Return to pot.) Stir in cream and maple syrup.

Ladle soup into wide shallow bowls. Serve with French Onion Toast Toppers and top with parsley.

French Onion Toast Toppers:

Preheat the oven to 425 degrees F (220 degrees C). Heat butter and olive oil in a very large skillet over medium-low heat until butter is melted, 1 to 2 minutes. Add sweet onions, shallot, salt, and pepper. Cook, covered, stirring occasionally, until onions are tender, 12 to 14 minutes. Increase heat to medium-high. Cook, uncovered, stirring frequently, until onions are golden brown, 3 to 4 minutes.

Reduce heat to medium. Stir in sherry and cook 2 minutes more. Add low-sodium beef stock and fresh thyme sprigs. Bring to a boil. Reduce heat and simmer until liquid is reduced and onions are very tender, about 5 minutes. Remove thyme and discard.

Meanwhile, arrange sourdough bread slices on a large baking sheet. Spread each slice with 1 teaspoon softened butter. Bake, turning once halfway through, until light brown, 8 to 10 minutes. Preheat the oven's broiler.

Top bread slices with caramelized onion mixture and shredded Gruyère cheese. Broil until cheese is melted, about 2 minutes.

Chili-Topped Potato Soup

Things Needed

3 pounds baking potatoes

1 pound lean ground beef

½ cup chopped onion

3 cloves garlic, minced

1 (15 ounce) can tomato sauce

1 (15 ounce) can chili beans

1 (1.25 ounce) package chili seasoning mix

1 cup low-sodium chicken broth

¼ cup butter

4 cups milk

1 cup buttermilk

1 teaspoon salt

½ teaspoon ground black pepper

1 ½ cups shredded white Cheddar cheese

½ cup sour cream

chopped fresh chives (Optional)

Preparation

Preheat oven to 425 degrees F (220 degrees C). Prick potatoes with a fork. Transfer to a 10x15-inch baking pan.

Bake in the preheated oven, turning once, until tender, about 1 hour.

Meanwhile, for chili, add ground beef, onion, and garlic to a large saucepan. Cook over medium heat, stirring to break up lumps, until meat is browned and onion is tender, about 10 minutes. Drain grease.

Add tomato sauce, chili beans, and chili seasoning mix to saucepan. Bring to a boil. Reduce heat to low and simmer, covered, at least 10 minutes to let flavors meld.

When potatoes are cool enough to handle, use a spoon to scoop potato pulp into large bowl. (You should have about 4 cups pulp). Discard skins. Add broth to bowl. Mash potatoes until smooth.

Melt butter in a 4- to 5-quart Dutch oven over medium heat. Stir in flour and cook, whisking constantly to make a light roux, about 2 minutes. Gradually whisk in milk, 1 cup at a time. Cook, whisking constantly, until lightly thickened. Stir in potato mixture, buttermilk, salt, and pepper. Cook, stirring frequently, until heated through, 3 to 5 minutes (soup will be very thick). Remove from heat and gradually stir in 1 cup cheese.

Divide soup among bowls. Top with chili, sour cream, remaining 1/2 cup cheese, and chives (if using).

Creamy Tortellini Soup

Things Needed

¼ cup butter

½ cup finely chopped onion

3 cloves garlic, minced

¼ cup all-purpose flour

3 cups low-sodium chicken broth

3 cups chopped broccoli

1 medium carrot, julienned

1 (9 ounce) package cheese tortellini

½ teaspoon salt

¼ teaspoon freshly ground black pepper

¼ teaspoon smoked paprika

¼ teaspoon turmeric

½ cup heavy whipping cream

1 cup shredded Colby cheese

Preparation

Melt butter in a Dutch oven over medium-high heat. Add onion cook until soft and translucent, about 5 minutes. Add garlic and cook until fragrant, about 30 seconds. Sprinkle flour over onion-garlic mixture. Stir to combine, until flour is incorporated.

Slowly pour in chicken broth, stirring to combine. Add broccoli, carrot, and tortellini. Season with salt, pepper, paprika, and turmeric. Stir to combine and reduce heat to medium. Cover and simmer until broccoli is tender and tortellini are cooked through, about 15 minutes.

Stir in cream and cheese until melted. Serve immediately.

Mulligatawny Soup

Things Needed

½ cup chopped onion

2 stalks celery, chopped

1 carrot, diced

¼ cup butter

1 ½ tablespoons all-purpose flour

1 ½ teaspoons curry powder

4 cups chicken broth

½ apple, cored and chopped

¼ cup white rice

1 skinless, boneless chicken breast half - cut into cubes

1 pinch dried thyme

salt and ground black pepper to taste

½ cup heavy cream, heated

Preparation

Melt butter in a large soup pot over medium heat. Add onions, celery, and carrot and sauté until soft, 5 to 7 minutes. Add flour and curry, and cook 5 more minutes, stirring frequently. Add chicken broth, mix well, and bring to a boil. Reduce heat and simmer for about 30 minutes.

Add apple, rice, chicken, thyme, salt, and pepper. Simmer until rice is tender, 15 to 20 minutes.

Just before serving, stir in hot cream.

Beef Barley Vegetable Soup

Things Needed

1 (3 pound) beef chuck roast

½ cup barley

1 bay leaf

2 tablespoons oil

3 carrots, chopped

3 stalks celery, chopped

1 onion, chopped

1 (16 ounce) package frozen mixed vegetables

4 cups water

1 (28 ounce) can chopped stewed tomatoes

4 cubes beef bouillon cube

1 tablespoon white sugar

¼ teaspoon ground black pepper, or more to taste

salt to taste

Preparation

Place chuck roast in a slow cooker. Cook on High until tender, 4 to 5 hours. Add barley and bay leaf during the last hour of cooking.

Remove meat; chop into bite-size pieces. Discard bay leaf. Set beef, broth, and barley aside.

Heat oil in a large stock pot over medium-high heat. Sauté carrots, celery, onion, and frozen mixed vegetables until tender, 5 to 7 minutes.

Add water, stewed tomatoes, beef bouillon cubes, sugar, 1/4 teaspoon pepper, and beef-barley-broth mixture. Bring to boil, reduce heat, and simmer 10 to 20 minutes.

Season with salt and pepper before serving.

Chinese Corn Soup

Things Needed

1 (15 ounce) can cream style corn

1 (14.5 ounce) can low-sodium chicken broth

1 tablespoon cornstarch

2 tablespoons water

1 large egg, beaten

Preparation

Combine corn and chicken broth in a saucepan. Bring to a boil over medium-high heat.

Mix together cornstarch and water in a small bowl or cup; pour into the boiling corn soup, and continue cooking for about 2 minutes, or until thickened.

Gradually add beaten egg while stirring the soup. Remove from heat and serve.

Roasted Acorn Squash Soup

Things Needed

2 acorn squash, halved and seeded

water, as needed

3 tablespoons unsalted butter

1 large sweet onion, chopped

1 large carrot, peeled and chopped

1 clove garlic, minced

3 ½ cups low-sodium chicken stock

¼ cup half-and-half

½ teaspoon ground nutmeg

½ teaspoon ground cinnamon

1 pinch salt and ground black pepper to taste

Preparation

Preheat the oven to 400 degrees F (200 degrees C).
Arrange squash cut-side down in a baking dish.
Pour enough water into the baking dish to cover
the bottom.

Bake squash in the preheated oven until easily
pierced with a knife, about 45 minutes. Remove
from the oven and cool until easily handled. Scoop
flesh into a bowl and set aside.

Melt butter in a pot over medium-high heat. Add
onion, carrot, and garlic; cook and stir until onion
has softened and turned translucent, about 5 to 7
minutes. Pour chicken stock into the pot; stir in
squash and simmer for 20 minutes.

Fill blender halfway with soup mixture. Cover and
hold lid down; pulse a few times before leaving on
to blend. Puree in batches until smooth and return
to pot.

Stir in half-and-half, nutmeg, and cinnamon; season with salt and pepper. Thin the soup with water if desired.

French Onion Soup Gratinée

Things Needed

4 tablespoons butter

2 large red onions, thinly sliced

2 large sweet onions, thinly sliced

1 teaspoon salt

1 (48 fluid ounce) can chicken broth

1 (14 ounce) can beef broth

½ cup red wine

1 tablespoon Worcestershire sauce

2 sprigs fresh parsley

1 sprig fresh thyme leaves

1 bay leaf

1 tablespoon balsamic vinegar

salt and freshly ground black pepper to taste

4 thick slices French bread

8 slices Gruyère cheese, at room temperature

½ cup shredded Asiago cheese, at room temperature

4 pinches paprika

Preparation

Melt butter in a large pot over medium-high heat. Stir in red onions, sweet onions, and salt. Cook, stirring frequently, until onions are caramelized and almost syrupy, about 35 minutes.

Stir in chicken broth, beef broth, red wine, and Worcestershire sauce. Bundle parsley, thyme, and bay leaf with kitchen twine; add to the pot. Simmer over medium heat for 20 minutes, stirring occasionally. Remove and discard herb bundle. Reduce heat to low; stir in vinegar and season with salt and pepper. Cover soup and keep warm over low heat while you prepare the toast.

Set an oven rack about 6 inches from the heat source and preheat the oven's broiler. Arrange bread slices on a baking sheet and broil, turning once, until well toasted on both sides, about 3 minutes. Remove from heat; do not turn off the broiler.

Arrange 4 large oven-safe bowls or crocks on a rimmed baking sheet. Fill each bowl 2/3 full with hot soup. Top each bowl with 1 slice of toasted bread, 2 slices Gruyère cheese, and 1/4 of the Asiago cheese. Sprinkle a little bit of paprika over the top of each one.

Cook under the hot broiler until bubbly and golden brown, about 5 minutes. Cheese will cascade over the sides of the crock and form a beautifully melted crusty seal as it melts.

Serve hot and enjoy!

Hamburger Soup

Things Needed

1 pound lean ground beef

5 cups water

1 (16 ounce) can diced tomatoes

1 (10 ounce) package frozen corn kernels

1 (8 ounce) can tomato sauce

1 cup chopped carrots

1 cup chopped celery

1 cup chopped onion

6 beef bouillon cubes

3 tablespoons ketchup

1 teaspoon dried basil

1 teaspoon salt

Preparation

Heat a large skillet over medium-high heat. Cook and stir ground beef in the hot skillet until browned and crumbly, 5 to 7 minutes. Drain and discard grease.

Combine beef, water, tomatoes, corn, tomato sauce, carrots, celery, onion, bouillon, ketchup, basil, and salt in a large stockpot; bring to a boil. Reduce heat and simmer for at least 1 1/2 hours.

Texas Cowboy Stew

Things Needed

2 pounds ground beef

2 pounds kielbasa sausage, sliced into 1/2 inch pieces

1 medium onion, chopped

2 cloves garlic, chopped

4 cups water

2 (15.2 ounce) cans whole kernel corn, with liquid

2 (15 ounce) cans pinto beans, with liquid

2 (14.5 ounce) cans peeled and diced tomatoes, drained

1 (14.5 ounce) can diced tomatoes with green chile peppers, with liquid

1 (10 ounce) package frozen mixed vegetables

4 medium baking potatoes, peeled and diced

2 teaspoons ground cumin

2 teaspoons chili powder

salt and pepper to taste

Preparation

Gather all Things Needed.

Cook ground beef in a large skillet over medium-high heat until crumbly but not yet cooked through, about 5 minutes. Add sausage, onion, and garlic; cook and stir until meat is no longer pink and onion is translucent, 5 to 7 minutes. Drain grease.

Transfer beef and sausage mixture to a large pot over medium-low heat. Add water, corn, pinto beans, diced tomatoes, diced tomatoes with chile peppers, and mixed vegetables. Stir in potatoes, cumin, chili powder, salt, and pepper.

Cover and simmer, stirring occasionally, for a minimum of 1 hour; the longer it cooks, the better it gets.

Hodge Podge

Things Needed

1 cup fresh green beans, trimmed and snapped

1 cup fresh wax beans, trimmed and snapped

1 cup diced carrot

1 cup diced turnip

4 cups water, or as needed to cover

¼ teaspoon salt, or to taste

2 cups cubed new potatoes

½ cup heavy cream (Optional)

6 tablespoons butter

½ cup water

1 tablespoon all-purpose flour

Preparation

Combine green beans, wax beans, carrots, and turnip in a stockpot; add water to cover. Stir in salt and bring to a boil. Reduce the heat and simmer for 30 minutes.

Add potatoes and simmer until tender, about 30 more minutes. Stir in cream and butter.

Whisk 1/2 cup water and flour together in a small bowl; mix into soup and cook until thickened, 3 to 5 minutes.

Mushroom Soup Without Cream

Things Needed

2 tablespoons butter

1 cup peeled and sliced carrots

1 cup sliced onions

1 cup sliced leeks (Optional)

½ cup sliced celery

2 pounds sliced fresh brown or white mushrooms

1 teaspoon fresh thyme leaves

6 cups chicken stock

salt and pepper to taste

½ cup chopped green onion

Preparation

Melt butter in a stock pot over medium heat. Add carrots, onions, leeks, and celery. Cook and stir until vegetables are tender but not browned, about 10 minutes.

Stir in mushrooms and thyme; cook until mushrooms are soft, about 5 minutes. Pour chicken stock into the pot; season with salt and pepper. Cover and simmer over low heat for 30 minutes.

Ladle into bowls; serve with green onions sprinkled on top.

Roasted roots & sage soup

Things Needed

1 parsnip, peeled and chopped

2 carrots, peeled and chopped

300g turnip, swede or celeriac, chopped

4 garlic cloves, skin left on

1 tablespoon rapeseed oil, plus ½ tablespoon

1 tablespoon maple syrup

¼ small bunch of sage, leaves picked, 4 whole, the

rest finely chopped

750ml vegetable stock

grating of nutmeg

1½ tablespoon fat-free yogurt

Preparation

Heat the oven to 200C/180C fan/gas 6. Toss the

root vegetables and garlic with 1 tablespoon oil

and season. Tip onto a baking tray and roast for 30 minutes until tender. Toss with the maple syrup and the chopped sage, then roast for another 10 minutes until golden and glazed. Brush the whole sage leaves with ½ tablespoon oil and add to the baking tray in the last 3-4 minutes to crisp up, then remove and set aside.

Scrape the vegetables into a pan, squeeze the garlic out of the skins, discarding the papery shells, and add with the stock, then blend with a stick blender until very smooth and creamy. Bring to a simmer and season with salt, pepper and nutmeg.

Divide between bowls. Serve with a swirl of yogurt and the crispy sage leaves.

LOW POTASSIUM SNACKS

No-Bake Energy Bites

Things Needed

1 cup rolled oats

½ cup miniature semisweet chocolate chips

½ cup ground flax seed

½ cup crunchy peanut butter

⅓ cup honey

1 teaspoon vanilla extract

Preparation

Stir oats, chocolate chips, flax seed, peanut butter, honey, and vanilla extract together in a bowl.

Roll dough into 24 balls with your hands. Arrange balls on a baking sheet and freeze until set, about 1 hour.

Thai Chicken Balls

Things Needed

2 pounds ground chicken

1 cup dry bread crumbs

4 green onions, sliced

1 tablespoon ground coriander seed

1 cup chopped fresh cilantro

¼ cup sweet chili sauce

2 tablespoons fresh lemon juice

oil for frying

Preparation

In a large bowl, mix together chicken and bread crumbs. Season with green onion, ground coriander, cilantro, chili sauce, and lemon juice; mix well.

Using damp hands, form mixture into evenly shaped balls that are either small enough to eat with your fingers, or large enough to use as burgers.

Heat oil in a large skillet over medium heat. Fry the chicken balls in batches until well browned all over.

Mango Salsa

Things Needed

1 mango - peeled, seeded, and chopped

¼ cup finely chopped red bell pepper

1 green onion, chopped

1 fresh jalapeño chile pepper, finely chopped

2 tablespoons chopped cilantro

2 tablespoons lime juice

1 tablespoon lemon juice

Preparation

Gather Things Needed.

Place mango, red bell pepper, green onion, jalapeño, cilantro, lime juice, and lemon juice in a medium bowl.

Mix Things Needed well to combine. Cover and let sit at least 30 minutes before serving.

Serve with chips.

Baked Tortilla Chips

Things Needed

1 (12 ounce) package corn tortillas

3 tablespoons lime juice

1 tablespoon vegetable oil

1 teaspoon ground cumin

1 teaspoon chili powder

1 teaspoon salt

Preparation

Gather all Things Needed.

Preheat oven to 350 degrees F (175 degrees C).

Stack tortillas in layers of 5 or 6. Cut through each stack to make 8 wedges. Arrange wedges in a single layer on rimmed baking sheets.

Combine lime juice and oil in a spray bottle or mister; shake until well mixed. Spray the tops of the tortilla wedges until slightly moist.

Combine cumin, chili powder, and salt in a small bowl; sprinkle mixture over the chips.

Bake in the preheated oven for 7 minutes.

Remove from the oven. Flip chips, then mist and season again.

Return to the oven, rotating the pans and switching racks. Bake, checking often to ensure they don't burn, until chips are lightly browned and crisp, 5 to 8 more minutes.

Remove from the oven and cool slightly before serving. Chips will crisp up more as they cool.

Enjoy with a side of salsa!

Banana Muffins with Sour Cream

Things Needed

1 cup all-purpose flour

1 tablespoon baking powder

½ teaspoon baking soda

¼ teaspoon salt

1 cup mashed ripe banana

¼ cup white sugar

¼ cup sour cream

1 egg

½ teaspoon vanilla extract

Preparation

Preheat the oven to 350 degrees F (175 degrees C).
Grease 12 muffin cups or line with paper muffin
liners.

Mix together flour, baking powder, baking soda, and salt in a large bowl.

Beat together banana, sugar, egg, and vanilla in a separate bowl. Stir in sour cream. Stir banana mixture into flour mixture until just combined. Scoop batter into the prepared muffin cups.

Bake in the preheated oven until a toothpick inserted into the center of a muffin comes out clean, 15 to 20 minutes. Let cool before serving. For best flavor, place muffins in an airtight container or bag overnight.

Fruit Leather

Things Needed

1 cup sugar

¼ cup lemon juice

4 cups peeled, cored and chopped apple

4 cups peeled, cored and chopped pears

Preparation

Preheat the oven to 150 degrees F (65 degrees C). Cover a baking sheet with a layer of plastic wrap or parchment paper.

In the container of a blender, combine the sugar, lemon juice, apple and pear. Cover and puree until smooth. Spread evenly on the prepared pan. Place the pan on the top rack of the oven.

Bake for 5 to 6 hours, leaving the door to the oven partway open. Fruit is dry when the surface is no longer tacky and you can tear it like leather. Roll up on the plastic wrap and store in an airtight jar.

Terrific Trail Mix

Things Needed

1 cup combination diced dried fruit, such as prunes, apricots, pears and apples

½ cup raisins and/or dried cherries or cranberries

1 ½ cups unsalted sunflower seeds

1 cup unsalted dry-roasted peanuts (or honey-roasted peanuts, chopped walnuts or unsalted almonds)

Preparation

Mix all. Makes 4 cups.

Super Easy Hummus

Things Needed

1 (15 ounce) can garbanzo beans, drained, liquid reserved

1 tablespoon lemon juice

1 tablespoon olive oil

1 clove garlic, crushed

½ teaspoon ground cumin

½ teaspoon salt

2 drops sesame oil, or to taste (Optional)

Preparation

Blend garbanzo beans, lemon juice, olive oil, garlic, cumin, salt, and sesame oil in a food processor; stream reserved bean liquid into the mixture as it blends until desired consistency is achieved.

Healthier Soft Oatmeal Cookies

Things Needed

1 cup butter, softened

½ cup white sugar

¾ cup packed brown sugar

2 eggs

1 teaspoon vanilla extract

1 cup all-purpose flour

1 cup whole wheat flour

1 teaspoon baking soda

1 teaspoon salt

2 teaspoons ground cinnamon

3 cups rolled oats

1 cup diced, pitted dates

Preparation

Beat butter, white sugar, and brown sugar with an electric mixer in a large bowl until smooth and creamy. Add eggs one at a time, mixing well after each addition. Mix in vanilla.

Combine flours, baking soda, salt, and cinnamon in a separate bowl; stir into creamed mixture. Fold in oats and dates. Cover and chill dough in the refrigerator for at least 1 hour.

Preheat the oven to 375 degrees F (190 degrees C). Grease 2 baking sheets.

Roll dough into walnut-sized balls and place 2 inches apart onto the prepared baking sheets. Flatten each cookie with a large fork.

Bake in the preheated oven until cookies are golden brown, 8 to 10 minutes. Cool cookies on the baking sheets for 5 minutes, then transfer to a wire rack to cool completely.

Fruit Dip

Things Needed

1 (8 ounce) package cream cheese, softened

1 (7 ounce) jar marshmallow creme

Preparation

Gather cream cheese and marshmallow creme.

Place cream cheese and creme in a medium bowl

Blend cream cheese and marshmallow creme with

an electric mixer until smooth and well combined.

Serve with fruit and enjoy!

Alabama Fire Crackers

Things Needed

1 ⅔ cups vegetable oil

2 (1 ounce) envelopes ranch dressing mix

3 tablespoons crushed red pepper flakes

1 teaspoon garlic powder

1 teaspoon onion powder

½ teaspoon black pepper

1 (16.5 ounce) package multigrain saltine crackers

Preparation

Place vegetable oil, ranch dressing mix, crushed red pepper flakes, garlic powder, onion powder, and black pepper in a 2-gallon resealable plastic bag. Seal the bag and squeeze with your hands until oil and spices are well combined.

Place crackers into the bag, seal, and turn the bag over to coat crackers with spice mix. Let sit for about 1 hour, then turn again. Repeat several times until crackers are well-coated with spice mix, then allow the bag to sit 8 hours to overnight. Remove crackers and serve.

Chocolate Cake Batter Hummus

Things Needed

1 (15 ounce) can chickpeas, drained and rinsed

3 tablespoons cocoa powder

3 tablespoons maple syrup

2 tablespoons water, or as needed

2 tablespoons tahini

½ teaspoon vanilla extract

1 pinch salt

Preparation

Combine chickpeas, cocoa powder, maple syrup, water, tahini, vanilla extract, and salt in the bowl of a mini food processor. Blend until smooth, scraping down the sides of the bowl. Add additional water, 1 tablespoon at a time, until hummus is smooth.

Sweet, Salty, Spicy Party Nuts

Things Needed

cooking spray

1 cup untoasted walnut halves

1 cup untoasted pecan halves

1 cup unsalted, dry roasted almonds

1 cup unsalted, dry roasted cashews

1 teaspoon salt

½ teaspoon freshly ground black pepper

¼ teaspoon ground cumin

¼ teaspoon cayenne pepper

½ cup white sugar

¼ cup water

1 tablespoon butter

Preparation

Preheat the oven to 350 degrees F (175 degrees C).

Line a baking sheet with aluminum foil and lightly coat with cooking spray.

Combine walnuts, pecans, almonds, and cashews in a large bowl. Add salt, black pepper, cumin, and cayenne; toss to coat.

Heat sugar, water, and butter in a small saucepan over medium heat. Cook until butter is melted and sugar is dissolved, about 1 minute. Slowly pour butter mixture over nuts and stir to coat.

Transfer nuts to the prepared baking sheet and spread into a single layer.

Bake nuts in the preheated oven for 10 minutes. Stir nuts to coat with warm syrup; spread out in a single layer. Return to the oven and bake until nuts are sticky and roasted, about 6 more minutes. Allow to cool before serving.

Banana muffins

Things Needed

2 large eggs

150ml pot natural low-fat yogurt

50ml rapeseed oil

100g apple sauce or puréed apple

1 ripe banana, mashed

4 tablespoon honey

1 tablespoon vanilla extract

200g whole meal flour

50g rolled oats, plus extra for sprinkling

1 ½ tablespoon baking powder

1 ½ tablespoon bicarbonate of soda

1 ½ tablespoon cinnamon

100g blueberry

2 tablespoon mixed seed, we used pumpkin, sunflower and flaxseed

Preparation

Heat oven to 180C/160C fan/gas 4. Line a 12-hole muffin tray with 12 large muffin cases. In a jug, mix the eggs, yogurt, oil, apple sauce, banana, honey and vanilla. Tip the remaining Things Needed, except the seeds, into a large bowl, add a pinch of salt and mix to combine.

Pour the wet Things Needed into the dry, mix briefly until you have a smooth batter, don't over mix as this will make the muffins heavy. Spoon the batter between the cases. Sprinkle the muffins with the extra oats and the seeds. Bake for 25-30 minutes until golden and well risen, and a skewer inserted to the centre of a muffin comes out clean. Remove from the oven, transfer to a wire rack and leave to cool. Store in a sealed container for up to 3 days.

Roasted carrot and whipped feta tart

Things Needed

large bunch of carrots with tops (about 800g)

2 tablespoon olive oil

1 tablespoon za'atar

2 tablespoon honey

125-150ml extra virgin olive oil

2 garlic cloves, roughly chopped

50g walnuts, roughly chopped

40g grated parmesan or vegetarian hard cheese

25g parsley, roughly chopped, plus whole leaves to serve

200g feta drained and crumbled (vegetarian, if needed)

150g Greek yogurt

1 lemon, zested

500g block puff pastry

1 egg, beaten

Preparation

Heat the oven to 200C/180C fan/gas 6. Trim off the carrot tops, discarding any tough stems, then set aside. Halve the carrots lengthways, tip into a roasting tin and toss with the olive oil and some seasoning. Roast for 25-30 minutes until tender and golden, stirring once or twice to ensure they don't stick. Stir in the za'atar and honey, and set aside.

Meanwhile, tip the reserved carrot tops and extra virgin olive oil into a food processor. Season and blitz, scraping down the sides occasionally until finely chopped. Add the garlic, walnuts, parmesan and parsley, and pulse until combined. Pour in another splash of olive oil, if needed. Transfer to a bowl and season to taste. Clean out the food processor, then tip in the feta, yogurt, most of the lemon zest and some seasoning. Blitz until smooth and creamy.

CHAPTER V: FINALLY!

Potassium, a vital mineral abundantly present in various everyday foods, plays a crucial role in maintaining optimal muscular function, particularly within the cardiac muscle. Despite its significance, many individuals fail to meet the recommended daily intake of 3,400 mg for males and 2,600 mg for females.

It is imperative to acknowledge that hypokalemia, a deficiency of potassium in the body, seldom stems solely from inadequate dietary intake. Factors such as fluid depletion, prolonged fasting, traumatic shock, medication usage, and underlying medical conditions like renal insufficiency can all contribute to disturbances in electrolyte balance.

The manifestations of potassium deficiency encompass a spectrum of symptoms, including weakness, fatigue, muscle cramps, aches, tingling sensations, cardiac palpitations, respiratory distress, gastrointestinal disturbances, and fluctuations in blood pressure.

Given the potentially severe consequences of potassium depletion, seeking medical attention promptly is paramount if one suspects a deficiency. Urgent medical intervention becomes imperative in the presence of abrupt alterations in respiratory or cardiac function.

While over-the-counter potassium supplements may seem like a convenient solution, self-administration is generally discouraged without professional guidance. Potassium chloride supplements, typically prescribed in doses ranging from 60 to 80 mmol per day, are commonly employed in managing mild to severe cases of hypokalemia, as they facilitate efficient restoration of potassium levels without the risk of rebound hyperkalemia.

However, it is essential to exercise caution, as potassium supplements have the potential to irritate the gastrointestinal mucosa, potentially leading to gastrointestinal bleeding or ulceration. Hence, it is advisable to consume them alongside meals and plenty of fluids to mitigate the risk of adverse effects.

Excessive potassium supplementation can precipitate hyperkalemia, a condition characterized by dangerously elevated blood levels of potassium, which can precipitate life-threatening cardiac arrhythmias and other serious cardiovascular complications. Therefore, the use of potassium supplements should be judiciously guided by medical professionals and closely monitored during administration.

Furthermore, individuals with specific medical conditions may necessitate prolonged adherence to a potassium-restricted diet, tailored to their unique circumstances. Regular consultations with a registered dietitian are indispensable for tracking progress, making necessary adjustments to dietary regimens, and ensuring optimal management of potassium balance.